THE
CAREGIVER

The Greatest Achievement
of my Career and in Life

TROY DONAHUE JACKSON

The Caregiver
© 2023 by Troy Donahue Jackson

Print ISBN: 978-1-66788-780-7
eBook ISBN: 978-1-66788-781-4

1st edition

Printed in the United States of America

Dedicated

To my mother, Gloria Jackson.

You gave me the gift of life, and

then I gave you the gift of a

caregiver

Everyone will someday need a caregiver.

This book will help current caregivers and those who are thinking about becoming one. If you know of anyone who needs this book, please pass it on to them, because someone is going through this with a family member. A friend, co-worker, church member, or someone else you socialize with is having this crisis with a loved one at this moment, because the need for caregivers is universal.

TABLE OF CONTENTS

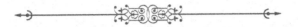

Introduction   1

Chapter 1: March 2020, the Height of the COVID-19 Pandemic   3

Chapter 2: The Sacrifice of Being a Caregiver   9

Chapter 3: The Financial Burden   15

Chapter 4: Hurricane Ida   17

Chapter 5: Contracting COVID-19 from the Physical Therapist   21

Chapter 6: The Upkeep of a Loved One   23

Chapter 7: Preparing Food as a Caregiver   25

INTRODUCTION

This book is about being a caregiver and what it takes to be one, first-hand from Troy Donahue Jackson, a proven caregiver for his mother, Gloria Jackson, as her only child and son. He has been taking care of his mother since he was in the twelfth grade when his dad passed away. This book will enlighten readers, in detail, about caregiver's responsibilities and the daily challenges they face. What it takes to be a caregiver, because being it requires selflessness, compassion, and, most important, love!

Troy Donahue Jackson gave up his corporate career as a marketing analyst to be a caregiver to his mother during the COVID-19 pandemic. His care-giving experience was complicated by Hurricane Ida, when they were without power for two weeks, as well as two cold days and nights when the power grid went down in the middle of the winter. Troy still cares for his mother. Troy continues to make sacrifices for his mother, and strives daily to be the best caregiver he can be for his critically ill mother, who has heart failure, respiratory failure, chronic obstructive pulmonary disease (COPD), poor circulation, high blood pressure, diabetes, lymphedema, and neuropathy with limited mobility issues. She is also on oxygen twenty-four hours a day.

CHAPTER 1:

March 2020, the Height of the COVID-19 Pandemic

On Sunday afternoon, March 31, 2020, Gloria Jackson was sitting on her front porch in her rocking chair at her home in New Orleans, Louisiana. She had several serious health problems at seventy-nine years old, but was managing them. After sitting on the porch for several hours to get fresh air after being in the house for so long due to pandemic lockdowns. Around 5:30 p.m., I noticed she had become incoherent and seemed to be about to lose conscious. I thought she was having a stroke, so I put her in my truck and rushed her to the nearest emergency room (ER).

COVID-19 was high at this time. I drove onto the hospital ramp and I was met by fully gowned, masked, and gloved nurses, who told me I couldn't come inside and they would call me in a couple of hours. I proceed back home, waiting on pins and needles for a phone call. Two hours later, I received a call from the hospital, telling me that my mom was in bad shape. She couldn't breathe on her own, and they asked for permission to put her on a ventilator. I gave them my permission, and also to resuscitate if needed. They put her in the critical care unit, on a ventilator, and gave her heavy sedation around the clock. The ER doctor called and told me that her Carbon Dioxide (CO_2) levels were 124, and normal levels are twenty to thirty-five; my mother's levels were four times that. At that time, her medical conditions included heart and repository failure, with atrial fibrillation. The hospital kept her on the ventilator for ten days. They did a COVID-19 test, and it came back negative. They kept her for three more days, and then sent her home by ambulance.

She had another attack, despite being on twenty-four hour oxygen at two liters. I called 9-1-1, and the ambulance returned her to the hospital with her CO_2 levels at 117. She was put back on the ventilator for seven more days in the cardiac care unit (CCU) for the second time in a month, but they let her come home after a week. She was home for two days, and I had to call the ambulance again, , G, once more. Gloria CO_2 level was ninety-seven this visit.

This time, a pulmonologist (lung specialist) recommended a BPAP machine, which is the cousin to the CPAP machine. The BPAP machine pulls the carbon dioxide from your body that your lungs are too weak to get rid of due respiratory failure. The lung specialist asked if she had one at home and if she had been diagnosed with this problem before. The nurse put the BPAP machine on that night, and the next morning her CO_2 level was seventy-six. The doctor extended her stay for two more days; the second day her CO_2 was fifty-four, and by the third day her CO_2 level was down to forty-eight. The BPAP has an adapter to hook up to her oxygen hose so she can receive both at the same time. In the morning, I remove the BPAP mask and put the oxygen only back on. I still perform this procedure seven days a week.

The hospital social worker asked me what nursing home I wanted my mother to go to, and I said, "Her house."

The social worker said, "Your mother will need twenty-four-hour, around-the-clock care."

My mother started crying and asked me not to put her in the nursing home. I visit her room in person and told her she was going home with me. This put a smile on her face.

The medical staff contacted a medical equipment company to set up at her home as a hospice with a motorized hospital bed, twenty-four-hour oxygen, a BPAP machine, bedside commode, nebulizer breathing treatment machine, and portable oxygen tanks for emergency use if the power went out.

Since she had been on the ventilator for twenty days, the tube hurt her throat and made it hard to swallow. She didn't want to eat anything, and was still incoherent from the Fentanyl and Propofol. I had to turn her over to keep her from getting bedsores and her skin breaking down. She was totally incontinent, and I had to use the bedpan for bowel movement daily, lifting her up and rolling her back and forth to change her diaper. Mom weighed 350 pounds and was very weak at seventy-nine years old. Today she is eighty-one years old.

In 2020, the doctors had given up on her, thinking she wouldn't last long. Neither God nor I gave up on her, and He has helped every day since March 2020. It hasn't been easy, but I endure and am still standing strong due to my faith. I give her love every day, and this is the best medicine you can give anyone, love.

The first thing I had to do was to fully detox her from the Fentanyl and Propofol from the ventilator. I started with soft baby food that she could swallow easily at first. This process lasted three months, then I added mashed potatoes, fresh and frozen vegetables, gelatin, multi-vitamins including B-12, Zinc, Vitamin D (5000 IU), and plenty of water to flush the medications out of her system. At her age and due to her poor health, her body couldn't get rid of them by itself, so I had to help her system out with this process because it would have taken a lot longer and she could have become dependent on these drugs in her system. Her diet included fresh green vegetables, and no processed, salty, sugary, or fried foods were in her diet.

CHAPTER 2:

The Sacrifice of Being a Caregiver

⟶ ❊❦❊ ⟵

Everybody talks a good game about what they would do for a family member, but they will give up after the first thirty days if they last that long, because it's too much and they don't want to give up their lifestyle, status, social life, and friends, so-called friends at that. All of the material things don't exist anymore because reality sets in and you are all by yourself with no help or support. Everybody runs from you because they are living their best life.

Remember, everyone gets old, that's a given, whether they're a CEO, doctor, lawyer, or politician. Everyday people need someone to take care of them one day, and that day will come sooner than you think!

There were lots of sleepless nights, since this was a twenty-four-hour job. I gave up my career and stepped out on faith, doing the right thing in my life. If my mother went to a nursing home, with the care they give, she wouldn't last a month because there is no love there, like a caring family member or loved one who cares. Love is the key and answer to everything in life, because that's what kept hope alive in my mother. She didn't give up and was determined to live because she saw my dedicated and unconditional love for her. My mother tells everyone that God and her son worked hard worked hard to keep her health stable, when everybody else turned their backs, both family and friends. They wouldn't bring my mother a glass of water, not that she needed it. They never offered anything out of courtesy after all she had done for them!

Remember love is courtesy and kindness in one. You find out the hard way who really cares when you are down and out and sick, and can't help yourself. But God doesn't count you out, and God is the only one who knows how to count! Caregiver, schoolteacher, police officer, and firefighter are at top of the list of tough jobs to perform on a daily basis. Those people are a special breed, and go beyond the call of duty! They are unsung heroes who receive no recognition, but are important. The caregivers are on the front line with no support. If I had the resources, I would fund all caregivers in the world.

The daily care of a loved one is a task that supersedes anything else in life. They first must have love in order to embrace the task at hand. When you love what you do with passion, it shows. Caregivers have the greatest traits and skills, because they have leadership, decision-making, and executive skills. Those skills are critical to their success in caring for a loved one. They have to be self-motivated and determined, with a winning attitude, to accomplish the daily tasks at hand. Organizational skills, timelines, and deadlines must be met when dealing with insurance companies, bills, medical professionals, and so on when caring for a critical-care loved one! I wear several hats on a daily basis, including doctor, nurse, dietician, and physical and occupational therapist, all wrapped up in one service. I perform all of the following duties each and every day.

- Eating
- Toileting
- Bathing
- Light Housekeeping
- Dressing
- Food Preparation & Storage

- Grooming
- Grocery Shopping
- Transferring
- Laundry
- Ambulation
- Medication Reminders

I test Gloria's blood sugar, blood pressure, breathing treatment, oxygen level, and heart rate; prepare the BPAP machine at bedtime and remove it at 6 each morning, every day. I assist with medicine, transfer her from bed to commode, deal with incontinence, dress and groom her, wash and dry clothes and bed linens, grocery shop, and cook three meals plus two snacks each and every day since March 2020. There's no time off or complaining because I enjoy what I do. Giving love to a loved one is giving them life, and I look forward to each day and am grateful and thankful that God has me as her guardian angel, taking care of her.

If a person has ten children, there is no guarantee that any of them will take care of their parents. Most people want material things and let their parents go to the dogs in a nursing home. They have no love for the people who brought them into the world and are the reason they are successful today! It is time to give back to your loved ones. Because by paying it forward, I look forward to someone taking care of me when I get old. Karma is real, that's why love is so important.

CHAPTER 3:

The Financial Burden

‑‑‑‑‑‑‑‑‑❧❧❧‑‑‑‑‑‑‑‑‑

B eing a caregiver comes at a price, because you are giving yourself to do the right thing in life and not worrying about status or income. The well being of your loved one is more important than anything!

Give them flowers while they are living, and there will be no guilt later on. The insurance doesn't cover everything; some medicines are not covered and neither are most over-the-counter items. Even some medical equipment is not covered. Gloria is on a fixed income, and it's hard and stressful! Take caution!

Caregiving is not for the weak! This is the biggest reason that people don't want to be a caregiver. They take the easy route, put their loved one in a nursing home, and forget about them. On my limited resources, I have to make sure that I'm on top of everything each month, such as the mortgage, home and flood insurance, real estate taxes, student loans, food, utility bills, and any other emergency expenses. I take care of these things twenty-four hours a day, 365 days a year. I have been doing this for three years and counting. My savings is gone, and I don't know how I do it, but God helps me make ends meet somehow. With faith and my good deeds, God provides for me out of nowhere for being a dedicated caregiver. The bottom line in being a caregiver boils down to time and resources, with inflation, the uncertain economy, supply chain issues, interest rates, high gas and light bills, the total cost of living, and everything else. People are living longer these days, and that must be taken into consideration as well. Giving my mom love makes her happy, and having dignity about herself keeps her going. If she was in a nursing home she wouldn't have lived this long. That's why I'm giving her flowers now, while she's living, because you only have one mother and one time to get it right. There is no second chance here. A person must first love themselves before they can love someone else; this is a requirement to be a good caregiver with both passion and compassion.

CHAPTER 4:

Hurricane Ida

H urricane Season for 2020 was more active and severe than any other season we have had, more than the normal amount. These hurricanes were back-to-back, causing more devastation, and recovery time was put on hold because you had prepared for the next one coming. And occurring during the COVID-19 pandemic made it more stressful and complicated.

We had Hurricane Laura, Hurricane Delta, Hurricane Zeta, and Hurricane Ida, which was the worst of them all. My mother's mobility is zero. We had the emergency evacuation team call us and wanted to take my mom to a gym/warehouse facility without the proper setup for hospice. My mother needed twenty-four-hour oxygen and BPAP, plus other things to accommodate her. I thanked them for offering their service, but I told them I was prepared to take care of her myself and had a three-week supply of necessities. Hurricane Ida was very powerful and knocked out the power grid for two weeks. I had food and water for four weeks to survive. I had a backup generator for the oxygen, BPAP, electric bed, lights, breathing machine, microwave, refrigerator, freeze, A/C, stove, weather radio, and washer and dryer, and we made it for the two weeks till the power came back.

I didn't miss a beat for Ida Hurricane. I had her enough medicine for four weeks. I was truly a Boy Scout, prepared for any and everything. We were safe and secure the whole time the storm was going on. No matter what area of the country you live in, you must be prepared for your area's weather.

I have some bad news to share with you. More than thirty patients died at the shelter that they wanted to take my mother because they didn't have the proper equipment in place due to the of influx of people, supply–and–demand issues, and poor advanced continuity planning.

The hospice and critical care patients were stuffed in like sardines in a can and they all perished. No, thank you I told them. My mother would have been one of that number. I keep her alive and well at all costs with the survival skills I learned in corporate America. The company that was responsible for the shelter was held accountable, but is facing a class-action lawsuit for deceased senior citizens. My mother and I made it without any problems, we finally got power after two weeks, and didn't miss a beat because we were prepared for the worst.

CHAPTER 5:

Contracting COVID-19 from the Physical Therapist

M y mother and I were both exposed to COVID-19 by the physical therapist who comes to our home to give my mother therapy. On December 15, 2020, my mother and I both tested positive. My mother is at high risk because she has several severe health issues. I prepared soup, tea, and coffee, and took vitamin D, zinc, cough drops, and ate all green vegetables. We drink a case of water a day, and Pedialyte with zinc. We also took 650 mg of acetaminophen and cough syrup, checked temperature and oxygen levels every three hours, and did twenty-one days in quarantine. The asked my mother how she survived the COVID-19 virus with all of her health problems. She told them, "God and my son, with a diet of no processed food, no pork or beef, no fried food, no salt or sugar. My son cooks my food from scratch with love."

She is still on the same diet today. I prepare three meals and two snacks a day and we drink plenty of water. We have fresh or frozen food only, such as chicken, fish, and turkey. I got her appetite back by cooking fresh every day and making sure she takes her vitamins. She still has mobility issues due to be being eighty-one years old now and with stage-three lymphedema, is still on twenty-four-hour oxygen and breathing treatments because her lungs are weak due to COPD with respiratory failure. I also give her love every day! That is a medicine also, by the way. It makes her happy and puts a smile on her face, even when she is in pain. This is what gets her through, along with God almighty.

CHAPTER 6:

The Upkeep of a Loved One

—⸱)———— ⚜ ————(⸱—

The upkeep of a loved one is very hard. The caregiver has to stay on top of everything, so there is no breakdown of the skin, keep the toenails clipped, grease and moisturize the hair and skin from top to bottom. Most people are weak, but you have to be mentally strong to be a caregiver, without a doubt! Anyone can talk a good game, but nobody wants to do or put in the work. This is my payback for what she has done for me.

All of my friends and family have run away from me, including my girlfriend. These are selfish people who have no compassion or understanding. Life is real, but karma is also real and comes back to bite you really hard! This is why I'm humble and stay the course for the Lord and my mother. He gives me the strength to carry on each and every day!

CHAPTER 7:

Preparing Food as
a Caregiver

T he diet of an aging and sickly person has to be clean due to medical issues. My mother has diabetes and high blood pressure. That means no sugar, no salt, and anything else that shouldn't be in her meal. Fresh and frozen fruit and vegetables are the main foods, and protein is a must in the daily diet plan. No processed or canned food at all, and fast food shouldn't be in the diet. Cooking a balanced meal every day will help support nourishment of the body and soul. This will give them strength and make a difference much more than fried foods.

Here are some non-starchy vegetables:

- Artichoke
- Onions
- Asparagus

- Salad Greens
- Bean sprouts
- Sauerkraut
- Beets
- Spinach
- Broccoli
- Squash (summer, yellow)
- Brussels Sprouts
- Tomatoes
- Cabbage
- Tomato Sauce
- Carrots
- Turnips
- Cauliflower
- Water Chestnuts
- Celery
- Zucchini
- Cucumbers
- Eggplant
- Greens (collard, kale, mustard, turnip)
- Mirliton
- Mushrooms
- Okra

With the proper diet, medicine, and rest will help improve both blood sugar and blood pressure. The most important thing is to make sure that you stay hydrated with plenty of water and stay away from sugary juice, soft drinks, and caffeine. This is hard to do, but is necessary for good health.

This is why I prepare and cook everything fresh. It is so important and does the body so much good. Constipation is a real issue when taking different medications, and you have to be proactive with the diet to eliminate this issue. You are what you eat is a true saying.

Giving yourself to help other people is a gift. Caregivers are so important in life and are unsung hero. The Bible says charity is the highest form of Love, signifying the reciprocal love between God and man that is made manifest in unselfish love of one's fellow man. This has caregiver written all over it, and this is why I chose to be a caregiver to my mother.

In conclusion, thanks to everyone for taking the time to read my book. I hope everyone has enjoyed it and has found some takeaways to better understand the daily challenges of what it takes to be a true caregiver.

Tell family, friends, and your social media contacts, too, about this book. Maybe it will help someone who is dealing with this that you don't even know.

Contact the author:

Troy Donahue Jackson

P O Box 15703

New Orleans, Louisiana 70175

504-390-8997

Email: thecaregiver@thebookcaregiver.com

GoFundMe: https://gofundme/84a34990

The support Gloria Jackson receive, is a reflection of the person.